HIV/AIDS
TAKE IT EASY
BUT
TAKE CARE

KIBOKO FRANÇOISE MACHOZI

1

www.savelife.co.za

CONTENTS

INTRODUCTION

It is my observation that all patients are very concerned about the condition of their health and always want to be properly informed.

As stated in one of my earlier books: "Your guide for a healthy life", it is a bit difficult for a patient to heed a doctor's instruction if he does not understand the reason.

There are many pamphlets that educate people on the prevention of HIV, but very few focus on how to help affected persons understand their condition in order to achieve targeted treatments.

This has informed my authoring this booklet with a view to helping people affected by HIV understand what HIV / AIDS is about, how it affects the human being's body and how to fight against it.

The aim is to help the affected individual understand that HIV is just a chronic disease like other chronic diseases and similarly be well controlled.

HISTORY OF HIV

HIV stands for **Human Immunodeficiency Virus** while **AIDS** stands for **Acquired Immune Deficient Syndrome.**

At the beginning HIV was known as a zoonotic infection, meaning infection among animals. The transmission was also through sexual intercourse but without inducing immune-deficiency to the host.

It is thought that the disease was transmitted to humans while slaughtering an infected animal.

In humans, the virus causes damage to the body's immune system leaving it vulnerable to diseases and there are basically two types of the HIV virus namely HIV 1 and HIV 2

HIV 1 was found for the first time in 1983 originating amongst the chimpanzee in Central Africa and has now spread all over the world.

HIV 1 is subdivided into two different groups:

Group M (major)
Group O (outlier)
Group N found in 1998 in Cameroon
Group P found in 2009 in a Cameroonian woman.

The group M constitutes the majority of HIV 1 infection in the world.
HIV 1 group M is subdivided into subgroups which takes alphabetic letters from A to K.

The group O is smaller,

HIV 2 was found for the first time during the mid 1980s, its origin is from the monkey in western Africa and the virus is restricted to Western Africa.

HIV 2 possesses five subgroups.[i]

TRANSMISSION MODE OF HIV

The virus infects an individual through five general ways:

1. Unprotected sex with an infected person which is the most common method of transmission of the disease.

2. Transfusion of blood from an infected person.

3. Sharing an infected needle or any sharp material from an infected person.

4. Infection occurring during the birth of a baby born from an infected mother.

5. An infected mother may also pass the virus to the baby by breast feeding.[ii]

HIV LIFE CYCLE

For easy comprehension, I may say there are three major stages in the HIV life cycle which are:

Step one: The HIV gain entry into the T4 cell through the CD4 receptor (antigen on the surface of the T4 cell).

Step two: The virus combine its elements to the T cell elements and infects the cell.

Step three: The virus uses the T cell (human being antibody) genetic material to produce new viruses, which will also infect other T cells and continue the cycle.

IMMUNE SYSTEM

The immune system is a system which protects the body against infection and is composed of cells called antibodies or white blood cells.

Antibodies are produced by the body once it notices the presence of an antigen which are proteins found on the surface of germs.

The following are types of antibodies:

1. Lymphocytes
2. Basophiles
3. Eosinophiles
4. Netrophyles
5. Monophyles
6. Macrophages

Lymphocytes constitute plus minus thirty percent of white blood cells, it fights viral infections as well as help other white blood cells fight bacterial and fungal infections.

There are two kinds of lymphocytes which are called B cells and T cells.

B and T cells are created in the bone marrow but T cells mature in the thymus gland (Lymphoid organ).

T cells are divided into three major groups namely:

a) Helper T cells or T4 or (CD4 cells). This kind of lymphocyte fights viral infections and helps other white blood cells fight bacterial and fungal infections.

b) Suppressor T cells also called T8 or CD8 cells stop the activity of other lymphocytes from destroying normal cells.

c) Killer T cells or cytotoxic T lymphocytes or CTLs recognize and destroy infected cells.

In this booklet, we will focus on the specific antibodies which are mostly affected in the case of HIV infection.

HIV infection damages the antibodies called lymphocytes T4 on which we find a glycoprotein called CD4 receptor and uses them to reproduce new strains of viruses. This condition renders the immune system weak and unable to protect the body from infections.

CD4: Cluster of Differentiation N°4

This is a bunch of protein that constitutes a T4cell receptor and through which HIV gains entry into the T cell (HIV life cycle, step one).

CD4 is a receptor for HIV in a human body. The normal CD4 varies between 600 to 1200 CD4 cells/ mm^3, the lower the CD4 cells count the weaker the body's resistance to diseases.

Once the CD4 is under 200 cells/ mm^3 a person is considered to have AIDS as in most cases the individual will suffer from opportunist infections.

Without ART (Antiretroviral treatment), CD4 cells will drop to an average of 100 cells/ mm^3 per year and once the CD4 cells is about fifty cells/ mm^3, the life expectancy of an individual may not exceed twelve months.

HIV does not kill directly but does affect the immune system which renders the body vulnerable to all manner of diseases and leads to death.[iii]

BLOOD TEST

Everybody should know his or her status and there are many blood tests that should be carried out in cases of HIV infection.

These tests are carried out for different reasons namely:

-Diagnosis,
-Evaluation of the immune system
-Evaluation of the level of viruses in the Human body.
-Evaluation of the status of different body organs before starting ART.
-Checking the presence of opportunist infections.

1. DIAGNOSIS

There are three ways through which HIV diagnosis could be made namely:

1. 1. DETECTION OF ANTIBODIES AGAINST HIV IN THE BLOOD PLASMA

The presence of antibodies against HIV in an individual's blood is proof that the person is infected by the virus.

Antibodies against HIV are identified in an infected person between six to twelve weeks of infection, but it can take up to six months for a human immune system to produce enough antibodies to test positive through some blood tests.

There are different blood tests capable of detecting the presence of antibodies against HIV, some of which are:

FIRST LINE TEST OR PRIMARY TEST

These tests are affordable, but have a high rate of wrong results.

A person suffering from other diseases such as syphilis, lupus or lyme disease may test positive to HIV while he is not infected.

These tests are carried out at the first position and all the positive results are confirmed by a confirmatory test as the percentage of wrong result is high. In a case of negative result a confirmatory test is not necessary but a second primary test must be conducted after a certain period of time according to the window period of a chosen test.

Amongst them we find:

- EIA: Enzyme immune assay.

- HIV ELISA: Enzyme linked immunosorbent assay.[iv]

SECOND LINE TEST OR CONFIRMATORY TEST

These tests are more accurate than the primary tests, but are more expensive.

They are conducted to confirm the first line tests which were positive. They are not done at the first position as they are expensive.

Included in this category are:

- Western blot assay
- Indirect immunofluorescent antibody assay
- A line immunoassay[v]

NB: A confirmatory test invalidates the result of a primary test. It means if the primary test was positive while the confirmatory is negative, it is proof that the primary test was a false positive.

1. 2. IDENTIFICATION OF HIV ANTIGENS IN THE BLOOD

An antigen is a protein that provokes the production of antibodies by the host immune system.

Protein P24 test detects the presence of the P24 proteins found on the surface of HIV and which provoke the production of antibodies to HIV by the host immune system.

This test is efficient from the first week of infection until the third as the virus replication is high at this period of time. It helps to diagnose HIV at its early stage when antibodies against HIV are not yet produced.

When the antibodies to HIV become detectable the P24 antigens become less detectable as they bind themselves to antibodies. At this time an antibody based test is recommended.

This test is useful in cases of rape, injury with an infected material, diagnosis of HIV to babies born from HIV positive parents and blood transfusion.

A negative P24 antigen may mean that a person is not infected but it also might indicate that the level of P24 antigen is lower than the detectable level of the test. In such case, a confirmatory test is requested.[vi]

1. 3. NUCLEIC ACID BASED TESTS

These tests detect the presence of the genetic material of the virus. They include:

- DNA PCR (viral load)
- RNA PCR

These tests are conducted for several reasons which may include:

1. An early diagnosis of the disease for example in a case of rape, injury with a needle from an HIV patient. It is also carried

out on children born from HIV positive parents under the age of eighteen months.

2. As a confirmatory test.

3. To evaluate the efficiency of the Treatment.[vii]

WINDOW PERIOD

A window period means a period before the body's immune system can recognize the presence of germs and produce specific antibodies against them or a time before the virus elements may be seen in a specimen.
It is a period that goes from the time of infection to the time when the diagnosis can be made.
It is the time before the diagnosis of the disease may be made.

This is why a doctor may request a second test to be conducted after a period of time according to the window period of a chosen blood test.

A first negative HIV test must be confirmed by a second HIV test and in such a case a primary test is repeated after a certain period of time.

There is no need to use an expensive test to confirm a primary negative HIV test unless the second one becomes positive in which case, a confirmatory test will be requested.

NB: A person is able to transmit the disease during window period.[viii]

2. HOW DO YOU MONITOR HIV INFECTION?

You monitor HIV infection by:

1. Evaluating the immune system,
2. Evaluating the level of viruses in a human being body,
3. Checking the presence of opportunist infections.[ix]

2. 1. EVALUATION OF THE IMMUNE SYSTEM

In a case of HIV infection the evaluation of the immune system is done by quantifying the CD4 cells as they are the most affected.

CD4 cells count shows to what extent the immune system is affected.
The normal CD4 cell count must be between 600 and 1200 cells/ ml, but in a case of HIV the CD4 cells can decrease until they disappear totally.

The lower the CD4, the weaker the resistance of the body to any disease and the higher the vulnerability and risk of death.

NB: Many countries initiate ART (antiretroviral treatment) once the CD4 cell drops below 350/ml as the risk of opportunist infections becomes higher at this stage.

2. 2. EVALUATION OF THE VIRAL LEVEL IN THE BODY.

Viral load estimates the number of the viruses in an affected body; it gives an idea about how far the disease has progressed.

Viral load may also be used to diagnose the disease at an early stage while the other tests may not have noticed the presence of the virus.

The viral load is a useful tool for the evaluation of the effectiveness of the treatment.

Before commencing ART, the viral load must be carried out and must be repeated regularly after the treatment has commenced to evaluate the efficiency of the treatment.

From the day a patient starts his ART the viral load must decrease until it becomes undetectable.

When the viral load is undetectable, it does not mean that the person is cured. The person will still be sick but the level of the viruses is lower than what the blood test may detect.
A person with an undetectable viral load must continue with his medications as if his viral load was detectable, otherwise the viral load will increase very quickly and a person may present resistance to the drugs he was taking.[x]

NB: In a case of undetectable viral load the risk of spreading the disease decreases to a certain level but not 100% as a person may still spread the disease even when the viral load is undetectable.

If the person is pregnant the risk of passing the disease to her baby is very low.

2.3. DIAGNOSTICS OF OPPORTUNIST INFECTIONS

Opportunist infections are those infections which may not easily affect an individual when his immune system is well built up (and even if they can affect a healthy individual, it will not be as serious as when compared to an immune suppressed individual), but those infections succeed when the immune system of an individual is compromised.

These categories of diseases include:

- Tuberculosis,
- pneumonia,
- Syphilis,
- herpes,
- Candidiasis and much more.

NB: There are also some conditions which are frequent among people living with HIV such as breast and womb cancer.

Test done to diagnose those opportunist infections are:

TB test: It is a test done to diagnose tuberculosis which may be diagnosed through sputum examination or by a chest X ray.

VDRL (RPR): Test done to diagnose syphilis.

Pap smear or Papanicolaou test to women: Test done to diagnose the cervical cancer.

Mammogram: Breast X ray/sonar done to detect breast cancer.

3.EVALUATION OF BODY ORGANS

Before commencing ART, the doctor would request for some blood tests in order to ascertain the status of various body organs which would influence the choice of ART.

It's important to note that some medications have side effects on the liver, others on the kidneys, others on the bone marrows and others could increase fat metabolism; such medications should not be given to any individual having even a minor liver problem or any of these other ailments, as it could worsen their condition.

SOME OF THE BLOOD TESTS ARE

Serum creatinine: This test is carried out to evaluate kidney function or the status of kidneys

Alt (SGPT): This blood test is carried out to evaluate the status of the liver.

Low density lipoprotein (LDL) is conducted to evaluate the level of the LDL in the blood stream.

FBC (full blood count): Is conducted to detect any blood synthesis problem.

The choice of ART will be made from these results.

PROPHYLAXY OF SOME OPPORTUNISTIC INFECTIONS

1. IMMUNISATION

Immunization may be given to HIV patients with a CD4 cells count higher than 200.

In cases of a CD4 cell count lower than 200, immunization must be avoided as it may lead to life threatening infection.

Common vaccines given to HIV patients are vaccine against:

    a. Flu
    b. Pneumonia
    c. Yellow fever
    d. Hepatitis B

2. TUBERCULOSIS PREVENTION

To prevent tuberculosis, a daily dose of isoniazid 300mg is given to all HIV patients with a positive tuberculin test for six months despite the level of CD4 cells count.

Precaution: Isoniazid may affect the liver and peripheral nerves and because of that the patient must report to the clinic any jaundice, nausea, vomiting and any nerve pains.

A daily dose of pyridoxine 25mg is associated to isoniazid to prevent nerve pain.

NB: The doctor may request a tuberculosis test to exclude TB before submitting a patient to isoniazid.

3. PROPHYLACTIC CO-TRIMOXAZOLE

To prevent pneumonia and other bacterial diseases, a doctor will request HIV patients whose CD4 count is below 200 cells/mm^3, to take 960mg of co-trimoxazole on a daily basis.

The treatment will be stopped only when the CD4 rises to 200 cells/ ml. [xi]

ANTIRETROVIRAL TREATMENT

Many things must be understood before starting antiretroviral treatment.

An individual must know very well what is ART, how does it work and how must it be taken in order to produce good results.

Once the ART has commenced it must not stop unless it was taken for prophylactic reasons.

The drugs must be taken at the same time every day and if a patient is sexually active it is recommended that a condom be used, as it would protect the patient not only from spreading the disease, but from recontamination which may introduce a new strain of virus that increases the risk of treatment failure.

The individual must be informed of the side effects and possible allergic reactions of chosen drugs, and all side effects and abnormal signs noticed must be reported immediately to the medical practitioner for follow up and investigation.

In a case of allergy the regimen will be changed as soon as possible until a suitable product is found for the particular patient.

Before submitting a person to ART the following blood tests should be carried out:

1. CD4 cells count
2. Viral load
3. Full blood count (FBC)
4. Cholesterol level
5. Kidney function
6. Liver function.

The choice of a suitable regimen is made according to the blood result.

The blood test is repeated six weeks after initiating the treatment, and every six months for the purpose of verification of the efficacy of the treatment and the effect of the chosen drugs on the body organs.

The viral load is a good indicator of treatment response and after six months the viral load should be undetectable.[xii]

TREATMENT FAILURE

Treatment failure or viral resistance is a condition in which the viral load does not decrease but increases despite the compliance of a patient to a suitable regimen.

The increase of CD4 cells differs from one patient to another, but usually there is a considerable increase of CD4 cells after four weeks of ART.

In some cases the CD4 cells count may not change despite the undetectable viral load. In such a case the doctor will not change the regimen.[xiii]

Is the use of condoms recommended even when both partners are HIV+?

- By having unprotected sex a person may get a new strain of viruses which may be resistant to the previous regimen.
- The couple will be exchanging viruses and it will be difficult for this couple to reach the treatment goals.

NB: When a person is on ART and is having unprotected sex, it will be like on one side he is decreasing the level of viruses and on the other side he is adding viruses. It will be difficult for this person to reach a level where his viral load becomes undetectable.

ANTIRETROVIRAL DRUGS

There is currently no cure for HIV, but there are antiretroviral drugs which are dispensed with the intention of:

    a. Decreasing viral load until it becomes undetectable,
    b. Increasing the CD4 cells count
    c. Reducing the frequency of diseases,
    d. Improving life quality despite the HIV
    e. Extending life expectancy
    f. Decreasing HIV transmission.

NB: These goals may be achieved only if the treatment is efficient and if the patient complies. For the treatment to be efficient it must be prescribed by a medical practitioner and must be taken as prescribed.

The viral load shows the efficiency of HIV treatment.

NB: There are many groups of ART which must be combined by three or four according to the case for a good result.

In order to increase the effectiveness of the treatment, pharmacists combine three to four products in one tablet as it is a bit difficult for an individual to swallow several tablets on a daily basis for a life time.

INTERACTION BETWEEN ART AND OTHER MEDICATIONS

There may be some medical interference between ART and other drugs. It could be that all drugs have the same side effects, it could also be that one drug decreases or increases the metabolic effect of another drug.

This is why it is recommended for patients submitted to ART to inform their medical practitioners about their status and show them all the medications they are taking. [xiv]

DIET AND EXERCISE

An HIV patient must eat a lot of fresh vegetable and fresh fruits to boost his immune system and to eliminate all the free radicals,
He must also consume high fiber food and seeds to decrease the level of cholesterol as there are some ART that promotes the accumulation of cholesterol.

Furthermore the patient must drink enough water, at least two liters per day as it is recommended for everybody.

The use of immune boosters is encouraged, but fresh vegetables and fruits are more effective as the body may assimilate all the ingredients easily unless the patient is not able to eat properly because of some condition like in a case of oropharyngeal candidiasis.

Exercise is good for everyone despite their status as it decreases bad cholesterol and increases the good cholesterol, it strengthens cardiac muscles and maintains the heart as it reduces stress and boosts the immune system.

NB: Stress weakens the immune system.

OPPORTUNIST INFECTONS

Opportunist infections are infections that occur because of immunodeficiency.

Infection that may not easily affect a healthy individual succeeds once the immune system is compromised.

Immune depression or immunodeficiency means the inability of the immune system to respond to attacks by germs because of the diminution of antibodies.

Causes of immune deficiency:

Immune deficiency could be caused by:

a. Some diseases like Cancer, Diabetes mellitus, Hypertension, Rheumatoid Arthritis, Asthma, Depression, HIV,
b. Some treatments such as Chemotherapy, Radiotherapy, Contraceptives made with high estrogen content and corticoids.

c. It could further be caused by conditions such as allergies, Malnutrition, pregnancy, Young age (babies), old age, stress, obesity[xv]

Whatever may be the cause of immune depression, opportunistic infections can be avoided. Your attitude toward your health plays a major role in the prevention of immune deficiency and opportunistic infections.

The following are lists of opportunistic infections:

- Tuberculosis
- Pneumonia
- Candidiasis
- Herpes zoster
- Genital herpes
- Seborrheic dermatitis
- Eosinophilic and bacterial folliculitis
- Fungal nails infection
- Diarrhea

The list is quite in exhaustive.

TUBERCULOSIS

Tuberculosis is a disease caused by mycobacterium tuberculosis or Koch bacillus.

Tuberculosis was first known as an endemic disease among animals which was later spread among human beings.

In Western Europe and America TB was discovered in humans since 1700 which further spread toward Eastern Europe, Asia South America and finally Africa from the 20th century.

In 1772 Benjamin Martin discovered that TB was infectious and might be transmitted by breath.

In 1882 Albert Koch discovered that TB was caused by a tubercle bacillus called mycobacterium tuberculosis which is why mycobacterium tuberculosis is called Koch bacillus.

He showed how to isolate the bacillus by doing sputum culture.

In 1919 Albert Calmette and Camille Guerin discovered a TB vaccine which is still currently useful and is called BCG (Bacille of Calmette and Guerin) from their names.

In 1921 the vaccine was used for the first time on humans.[xvi]

TUBERCULOSIS TRANSMISSION

Mycobacterium tuberculosis is emitted while coughing, sneezing, laughing, talking and even breathing, with transmission achieved by breathing contaminated air.

An individual may also contract TB by touching infected sputum.

For TB to be transmitted to another person there are some conditions which must exist:

a. The presence of an infected and non treated person
b. The receiver must be suffering from an immunosuppressant condition like malnutrition, Pregnancy, HIV, stress, depression, diabetes mellitus, cancer...
c. The source and the receiver must be sharing a room for long hours during the day or must be sleeping together for a long period e.g. people working together, people sharing the same house...
d. During winter TB transmission is easier than during summer because in summer windows and doors remain open for hours; people are outside most of the time but in winter everybody is inside the house maybe the whole day and windows and doors are always closed.[xvii]

TB STAGES

PRIMARY INTECTION

It is termed primary infection when a person is exposed to mycobacterium tuberculosis for the first time.

The body's immune response develops in four to six weeks after primary infection and may eliminate totally the infection but in some cases some bacilli maybe resistant to the immune response and in such a case, an individual may develop the disease after some months or years.[xviii]

ENDOGENOUS REACTIVATION

Once the immune system is compromised, the bacilli that are resistant begin to duplicate and the host develops the disease.[xix]

EXOGENOUS REACTION

This occurs when an individual catches a second strain of mycobacterium tuberculosis which makes stronger the previous one and develops into TB disease.[xx]

TB SYMPTOMS

At the beginning of infection the disease is asymptomatic but after a while the following symptoms appear:

1. Cough
2. Fever
3. Night sweating
4. Loss of appetite
5. Loss of weight
6. Loss of energy.[xxi]
7. Coughing up blood, chest pain and short breath may be present.

The disease is contagious from the time the individual begins to cough.

DIAGNOSIS OF TB

TB SPUTUM TEST

The TB sputum test may be done:

1. To diagnose TB.
2. To check if the patient is totally healed after a correct Tb treatment.

NB: For accurate results sputum TB test must be conducted twice or three times.[xxii]

TB CULTURE

TB culture is recommended:

1. When the patient presents all the TB symptoms but the sputum TB tests remain negative,
2. When the doctor think about extra pulmonary TB.
3. In cases of resistance to the TB drugs, for a purpose of sensitivity and choice of suitable drugs.

Principle of TB culture

Sputum is put in an environment suitable for TB bacillus to duplicate, after some days or weeks, that sputum is examined to diagnose the disease.

From this process the laboratory professionals expose those germs to different TB medications to check the sensitivity of the TB bacillus. [xxiii]

CHEST X RAY

Chest X- ray is made when all three sputum TB tests remain negative while all the TB symptoms are present.

TUBERCULIN TEST

Tuberculin test is used to diagnose a dormant TB especially in children.

The principle of the tuberculin test consists in injecting a PPD (purified protein derivate) into the skin and forty-eight to seventy-two hours later the body immune system will react to the PPD.

As a result an induration will develop on the injection area and the diameter of the induration will determine if the test is positive or negative.

For a non HIV patient a diameter bigger than fifteen millimeters is considered as positive while a diameter smaller than fifteen millimeters is considered as negative.

For an HIV patient a diameter bigger than four millimeters is considered as positive and a diameter smaller than four millimeters is considered as negative.
A positive tuberculin test indicates TB infection but not always a TB disease.[xxiv]

EXTRA PULMONARY TB

This is tuberculosis which develops outside the lungs such as:

1. TB of upper respiratory tract:

2. TB of epiglottis, larynx and pharynx.

3. TB of the mouth, tonsils and tongue
4. Military TB
5. Lymph nodes TB
6. Pleural TB
7. Genito urinary TB
8. Skeletal TB
9. Central nervous system TB
10. Abdominal TB
11. Pericardial TB
12. Adrenal TB
13. Cutaneous (skin) TB and subcutaneous (abscess) TB
14. Pott disease

TUBERCULOSIS PREVENTION

To prevent TB from spreading we have to:

1. Immunize children against TB (BCG) at birth.
2. Eliminating the source: Every person coughing for more than two weeks must be tested for TB and if the

person is affected, he must be treated properly.

NB: Once the person is on medication for two weeks he may not transmit the disease anymore, but the person is still sick and must therefore complete his treatment.

3. Avoid promiscuity,
4. Open windows even during winter to receive fresh air and dilute the concentration of mycobacterium tuberculosis.[xxv]

5. Isoniazid daily dose
In a case of HIV, Isoniazid is recommended to all patients with a positive tuberculin test but without any symptom of TB.

NB: Before starting the prevention regimen a liver function test must be done as isoniazid may be toxic for the liver.

The recommended dose is: isoniazid 5mg/kg (maximum 300mg per day) for 6 months.[xxvi]

Keep to your doctor's appointment in order to initiate ART once your CD4 cells count drop below 350 cells/mm³.

TB TREATMENT

Consult your nearest clinic for diagnosis and treatment.

For good results the patient should comply with the doctor's appointment in order to start ART once CD4 cells count goes below 350 cells/mm³ inclusive of healthy eating habit
.

Actually a six month TB regimen comprises of an association of four products namely:
  a. Rifampicin
  b. Isoniazid
  c. Ethambutol
  d. Pyrazinamide

A supplement of vitamin B6 is associated to the treatment to avoid the neurological side effects of isoniazid.

NB: In a case of resistance to the tuberculostatics (tuberculosis drugs) the treatment may be prolonged for up to 18 months.

PNEUMONIA

This is an inflammatory disease of the lungs characterized by the production of fluids.

CAUSES

Pneumonia may be caused by bacteria, viruses, fungi, parasites or chemicals.

Physical injuries to the Lungs may also cause pneumonia.

PROCESS OF LUNGS CONTAMINATION

a. Germs may reach lungs by inhalation of airborne's droplets,
b. While vomiting a person may inhale some germs from the digestive tract,
c. Germs may also reach the lungs via the blood stream when there is an infection somewhere else in the body, germs may be moving around and reach the lungs.

Once germs reach lungs, they invade the cells lining the airways, a process that may lead to cells death.

In response, the immune system activates some chemicals which make glands to produce fluids into the lungs thereby causing more lung damage.
Both germs and immune response to the infection are responsible of the symptoms.[xxvii]

SYMPTOMS

Symptoms for pneumonia are:

1. Productive cough with yellowish or greenish phlegm.
2. In some cases patients may cough up blood.
3. Chest pains
4. Short breath
5. Fever
6. Nausea and vomiting
7. Joints pains, muscles pain.

8. Blueness of the skin (lack of oxygen)
9. Headache
10. Fatigue
11. Sweating
12. Abdominal pain and diarrhea may be present in some cases especially in children.

DIAGNOSIS

The diagnosis of pneumonia is made by

- Chest x rays
- Blood tests
- Sputum (phlegm) culture.

PREVENTION

Adequate HIV treatment may decrease the risk of developing pneumonia and if the CD4 cells count is below 200, the doctor will prescribe a daily dose of co-trimoxazole 960mg until the CD4 cell count rises to 200 cell/mm^3.

There is the further need to desist from smoking in the case of smokers, smoking damages the lungs and weaken the immune system through the generation of free radicals.

Immunization against bacterial pneumonia and haemophilus influenzoe is necessary as haemophilus influenzoe can be complicated by viral pneumonia which can be further complicated by a bacterial pneumonia.[xxviii]

TREATMENT

The affected individual needs to consult the nearest clinic or doctor for diagnosis and treatment.

Generally the following procedure is observed in treatments for pneumonia:

1. Antibiotherapy
2. Fluid intake
3. Rest

In a case of viral pneumonia an appropriate antiviral will be added to the treatment.

PROGNOSIS

If an individual is committed to a good regimen, the disease may be cleared within two to four weeks but viral pneumonia may last longer.

Pneumonia may lead to septicemia (Generalized infection of blood).

Patients suffering from pneumonia develop short breath which will change the appearance of their skin to blue because of lack of oxygen. If there is no appropriate supply of oxygen death may be the final result.

COMPLICATIONS

1. A collection of fluid may be seen in the space surrounding the lungs (pleural cavity) a condition called pleurisy.

2. In some cases germs may infect this fluid and lead to emphysema and in such a case, drainage may be needed as antibiotics does not penetrate well into the pleural cavity.

3. Lungs abscess

4. Septicemia (a generalized infection of blood).

5. Death

Pneumonia is a major cause of death worldwide. [xxix]

ORAL AND ESOPHAGEAL CANDIDIASIS

Every person has candida albicans (the germ that causes candidiasis) in the digestive tract but these are not harmful until the individual's immune system is compromised.
.

Oropharyngeal candidiasis is common in people infected by HIV especially those with a CD4 cells count below 200 cells.

Candidiasis can also affect the esophagus leading to esophageal candidiasis which is characterized by a difficulty in swallowing food because of pain.

SYMPTOMS

OROPHARYNGEAL CANDIDIASIS

Lesions may be seen on gums, on the hard or soft palate, on the tongue, under the tongue and pharynx.

According to the appearance, candidiasis trash may be called:

Pseudomembranous: painless creamy white plaque on the tongue, gums, palate...

Erythemateux: Flat red spot at the posterior part of the tongue, gums, hard or soft palate,

Angular cheilitis: fissure or redness at one or both corners of the mouth.

NB: Chelitis may also be the result of:

- Riboflavin deficiency
- Allergic manifestation
- Bacterial infection

Other symptoms of candidiasis include:

- Unusual taste in the mouth
- Hypersensitivity of the tongue
- Loss of appetite[xxx]

ESOPHAGEAL CANDIDIASIS

This is evidenced by:

- Difficulty of swallowing food,
- Sensation of a blocked throat,
- Nausea, vomiting and loss of weight.
- Retrosternal pain

All the symptoms of oro-pharyngeal candidiasis may also be present.

DIAGNOSIS

a. Clinical examination,
b. Smear of the product of the lesion,
c. Culture and sensitivity is needed in the case of resistance to a first line therapy.
d. In a case of esophageal candidiasis endoscopy may be needed especially when the disease delays.

TREATMENT

PREVENTION

1. The HIV+ patient must ensure consistent compliance with the doctor's appointment for introduction to the ART once the CD4 cells count drops below 350 cels/mm^3,
2. Brush the mouth daily and gargle it with salty water after each meal
3. Eat healthy in order to boost their immune system.
4. Eat fresh garlic on a daily basis as it has antifungal effects.
5. Take milk and yogurt that have acidophilus bacteria which is a saprophyte bacteria that fight fungus and other pathogen bacteria.
6. Avoid sugar rich food as the germs that cause candidiasis (Candida Albicans) like sugar.
7. Avoid alcohol consumption as it converts into sugar and promotes candidiasis.

8. Exercise as it releases stress and boost your immune system.

CURATIVE TREATMENT

Consult the nearest clinic or doctor for diagnosis and treatment as the doctor will prescribe general antifungal drugs and a local antifungal cream.

NB: ART improves the condition.

Patient education:

- Patients must brush teeth using a soft tooth brush after every meal.
- They must remove teeth prosthesis if any and rinse the mouth very well before applying local antifungal cream.
- They have to avoid meal just after applying the product.
- They must avoid spicy and hot food[xxxi]

HERPES ZOSTER OR SHINGLES OR ZONA

This is a disease caused by a virus called varicella zoster and characterized by painful blisters limited to one side of the body.

The initial infection causes an acute short lived disease called varicella or chicken pox which upon recovery the virus remains in the body without causing any harm to the host. Once the immune system is compromised, the same virus rises again and causes shingles.

SYMPTOMS

- Malaise,
- headache,
- fever,
- burning sensation,
- sharp pains,
- itching,
- oversensitivity and sometimes numbness.

Upon infection and within three weeks, characteristic blisters will be present at one side of the body and never both sides.

DIAGNOSIS

The diagnosis is made clinically.

When blisters delay to develop the diagnosis of herpes zoster may be difficult and in such cases blood tests will be carried out.

NB: Herpes zoster may be seen only in people who suffered from chicken pox in the past.

A person suffering from chickenpox or herpes zoster can spread the disease from the time he or she develops blisters, till the time the blisters dry up.

.

Direct contact with chicken pox or herpes zoster blisters may spread the disease if the receiver has never suffered from chicken pox or never had a chicken pox vaccine administered. This individual will then develop chicken pox.

PREVENTION

1. Zostavax: Immunization against varicella zoster virus.

2. Diet rich in fibers, vitamins and minerals to boost your immune system.
   Exercise as it releases stress and boost your immune system.

If an individual is HIV+, he or she should ensure compliance with their doctors' appointment in order to initiate ART once their CD4 cells count drop below 350clls/mm^3.

TREATMENT

Patients should consult the nearest clinic for diagnosis and treatment and in most cases a doctor would prescribe:

a. Local and general pain killers.
b. Oral steroids.
c. Antiviral drugs

ART improves the condition.[xxxii]

GENITAL HERPES

Genital herpes is a sexually transmissible disease characterized by painful blisters on the private part that ulcerates and heals.

SYMPTOMS

1. Fever,
2. lack of appetite,
3. malaises,
4. presence of inguinal lymph nodes,
5. formation of painful blisters at the private part which ulcerate later,
6. vaginal discharge,
7. bleeding vagina,
8. pain on passing urine.

DIAGNOSIS

Biopsy

PREVENTION

Herpes simplex or genitalis as other STD can be avoided by:

a. A proper use of condoms,
b. Faithful monogamic relationship
c. Abstinence from sexual intercourse.

TREATMENT

Consult your nearest clinic or doctor for diagnosis and treatment as a doctor should prescribe:

1. Local and general pain killers.
2. Antiviral treatment.
3. In a case of recurrence the doctor may request to repeat the same treatment.
4. Spermicidal cream ameliorates the condition and stops the process.

PROGNOSIS

1. herpes genitalis may lead to cancer.
2. necrosing cervicitis sometimes caused by herpes genitalis may looks like stage 2 squamous cancer cells.
3. Herpes genitalis may lead to miscarriage, stillborn and may be the cause of neonatal death.[xxxiii]

SEBORRHEIC DERMATITIS

This is the inflammation of sebaceous glands characterized by:

1. an overproduction of sebum,
2. itchy skin,
3. presence of lesions on the skin,
4. formation of plaques over the affected skin,
5. loss of air and reddish skin affecting hairy areas (face, eyelids, ears, around the nose, scalp, axilla, upper trunk and groin).

This condition can be caused by:

1. A dry skin.
2. A yeast infection.
3. Stress,
4. Fatigue,
5. Heat,
6. Lack of proper skin hygiene,
7. Obesity and immune deficiency are trigger factors[xxxiv]

PREVENTION

1. Comply with all doctor's appointments in order to initiate Art once CD4 cells count drop under 350cells/mm^3
2. Eat healthy to boost your immune system.
3. Exercise in order to release stress and boost your immune system.
4. Keep your body and skin clean.
5. Avoid over sweating

TREATMENT

Consult your nearest clinic or doctor for diagnosis and treatment as the doctor may prescribe:

a. A local steroid cream.
b. Avoid soap and keep the skin moist.

The use of ART improves the condition.[xxxv]

EOSINOPHILIC AND BACTERIAL FOLLICULITIS (PIMPLES)

This is the presence of itchy papules or pustules mostly located in the follicles of hair. This condition is frequent in people living with HIV with a CD4 count lower than 200 cells/mm³; it is also frequent in other cases of immune deficiency.

PREVENTION

Patients must ensure compliance with all doctor's appointments in order to initiate Art once CD4 cells count drop under 350 cells/mm³

TREATMENT

Consult your nearest clinic or doctor for diagnosis and treatment as the doctor will prescribe:

1. Local steroid ointment
2. Antibacterial cream

ART improves the condition.^{xxxvi}

FUNGAL NAIL INFECTION

This condition is characterized by:

a. A swollen, reddish, painful nail bed and separation of the affected nail from the bed nail.
b. White discoloration of the proximal part of the nail plate with thickening.
c. The nail's color which may turn white, black, yellowish or greenish.
d. Toes nails which are more affected than fingers.

The infection start on the skin and if it is not well treated it spread to the nail.

CAUSE

- Immunodeficiency
- The wearing closed shoes for long hours as they will produce sweat,

- Regular damage to your nails or to your toes.

PREVENTION

a. The patient should comply with the doctor's appointment in order to start ART once CD4 cells count goes below 350 cells/ mm³.
b. Aerate your feet regularly in order to prevent them from sweating.
c. Avoid nails trauma and treat well all injuries noticed on your toes.

TREATMENT

Consult the nearest clinic or doctor for diagnosis and treatment as the doctor will prescribe:

a. Antifungal tablets for one month or two to three months for toe nails.
b. Avoid alcohol during therapy because some antifungal tablets increase the level of alcohol in the blood.[xxxvii]

DIARRHEA

This is the frequent passing of liquid stools which may be associated with vomiting or not, and may lead to dehydration.

CAUSE

- Infection
- Ingestion of a toxin
- Stress and emotion
- Allergies

TREATMENT

Consult your nearest clinic or doctor for treatment:

- Metoclopramide if the diarrhea is associated with vomiting.
- Oral rehydration fluids
- Loperamide to stop the diarrhea
- Elimination of the cause.

PRAYER

1. Thank God for the gift of life because the bible says there is expectancy for those who are still alive.
2. Thank him for the privilege he gave you to know your status. Other people did not know their status and are now dead, at least you know your status and you can do something about it by His grace.
3. Forgive the person who passed the disease to you even if you do not know him or her.
4. If you are not able to forgive him ask God to give you the grace to forgive, remember there is liberating power in forgiveness. When you forgive someone, you are doing justice to yourself because you are liberating yourself.

   Remember that you are also a sinner and you need forgiveness from God. How would you expect God to forgive you if you do not forgive others?

5. Ask God to forgive all your sins. If you are responsible for your condition ask Him to forgive you because you did not protect the temple of the Holy Spirit, as the bible says that your body is the temple of the Holy Spirit.

6. Ask God to forgive you because you passed the disease to others.

7. Pray for those people whom you passed the disease to, so that the grace of God will be with them.

8. If you are a victim of the disease, forgive your spouse. Do not avenge yourself, the bible does not recommend revenge but recommends forgiveness. Remember that only God can avenge you.

Believe in your prayer because the bible says "if you acknowledge that you have sinned and repent with all your heart, he is just and faithful to forgive you."

9. Pray for the grace of God to be up on you.
10. Pray now according to your faith. Remember that the Almighty God is the God who can heal even from incurable diseases like HIV/AIDS and much more.

Remember John 14:13 says "whatever you may ask from God in the name of Jesus Christ, it will be given to you."

Believe in your prayer and thank God.

CONCLUSION

HIV/AIDS is just a chronic disease like hypertension, Diabetes mellitus and much more.

Everybody should know his or her status and once you know your status take a decision to live a positive life.
If you are HIV negative it is very good news but do not forget that many of those affected by HIV were once HIV negative, it means you too may be HIV positive if you do not make the right decision.

It is very easy to change your status from HIV negative to HIV positive and currently the reverse is impossible except by God's grace.

If you are HIV positive, it is not the end of the world, life is precious. Do not allow HIV to destroy your happiness and your life.

You have power over HIV and you may destroy it by taking a decision to pray, to Stay positive, follow your doctor and counselors advice and comply with all the clinic appointments.

No disease has an ability to kill a human being unless you give it that power or if it is your time to die, God is the only one who may give or take away life from someone.

If it is your time to die you will, HIV or not and if it is not your time to die you will not die even when you are HIV positive unless you choose to die by rejecting health professional advices. Diseases are only a way of dying.

Please note that every day there are people dying from different causes and not only from AIDS. Some die from other diseases, car accidents while others just die when they are asleep.

For example when you are going to Cape Town you may go by plane, train or by bus, whatever the transport used you will end up in Cape Town, but on different times and in different conditions. The person who took a plane will arrive early and he will not be tired but the one who took a train or a bus will arrive late and he will be tired.

It is the same with death, everybody will die one day but at different times and from different conditions, some by car accident other by diseases, others just while they are sleeping.

If you follow your doctor's instructions you may live a normal life and have a long life even when you are HIV positive .If you do not take your life seriously you may die even when you are HIV negative.

Many people are devastated when they hear news that a relative or friend is HIV positive, they think they will have to bury him or her soon, but a surprise may be in store when the fellow makes a good decision and they don't, they may find themselves being buried by the fellow who is HIV positive.

In the book of Genesis 1:28 God gave to human beings authority over everything.

BE POSITIVE, FOLLOW THE HEALTH PROFFETIONAL'S ADVICE AND RESPECT YOUR CLINIC APPOINTMENTS.

GOD BLESS YOU

[i] Eskom, the integrated of TB, HIV and STD in the primary health care setting for doctors, section 2, page 10
Avert, history of AIDS up to 1986, found at www.avert.org/history of AIDS up to 1986
Avert, international HIV and AIDS charity, HIV types, subtypes groups and strains found at www.avert.org/hiv types
[ii] Public health-seatle and king country, how HIV is transmitted found at www.kingcountry.gov>public health home>communicable diseases and immunization>HIV/STD program>basic info on HIV/AIDS
[iii] Dr Leon Regensberg and Memela M Makiwane(Ed), 2009, AFA Clinical guide lines, pharmacy direct, page: 45
www.webmd.com/HIV AIDS/CD4 count
www.aidsmap.com/cd4 cell count

www.wbhealth.gov west Bengal, state prevention and control society,HIV/AIDS

www.thebody.com :The complete HIV/AIDS resource, What does CD4 stand for

www.hivaidsressource.org Health 24,The integration between viral load, CD4 cell count and disease progresstion, 21 july 2012.

[iv] www.about.com sexually transmitted diseases (STD), how does the doctor tests my blood?

MedlinePlus, Elisa/Western blot tests for HIV

WebMD,HIV and AIDS health center, Screening tests for HIV diagnosis and treatment found at www. webmd.com/.../HIV/AIDS sceening

[v] www.livestrong.com confirmatory tests for HIV

www.cdc.gov Act against AIDS for professionals, what is a confirmatory test?

www.aidsmap.com , Nam aidsmap, HIV transmission and testing, confirmatory tests

[vi] Lab tests online, p 24 antigen

www.aidsmap.com Nam aidsmap, HIV transmission and testing, p24 antigen

HIV insite, Nlel Constantine,phD, university of Maryland school of medicine, HIV viral antigen assays, sep 2001

[vii] AIDSinfo, testing for HIV

STOPAIDS, time it takes to test positive

[viii] Eskom, the integrated of TB, HIV and STD in the primary health care seting for doctors, section 2, page 48-52

[ix] Eskom, the integrated of TB, HIV and STD in the primary health care seting for doctors, section 2, page 73-87

[x] Michael Carter, Greta Hugshson, Nam AIDSmap, viral load,

[xi] Dr Leon Regensberg and Memela M Makiwane(Ed), 2009, AFA Clinical guide lines, pharmacy direct, page: 13-15.

[xii] Health24, antiretroviral treatment, found at www.health 24.com/Medical/HIV-AIDS

AIDSinfo, Clinical Guidelines Portal, Guidelines for the use of Antiretroviral Agents in HIV-1 infected Adults and

Adolescents found at
www.aidsinfo.nih.gov>home>guidelines>Adults and
adolescents ARV Guidelines.
[xiii] Dr Leon Regensberg and Memela M Makiwane(Ed), 2009,
AFA Clinical guide lines, pharmacy direct, page: 52
AIDSinfo, HIV/AIDS Health topics, treatment failure

[xiv] Dr Leon Regensberg and Memela M Makiwane(Ed), 2009,
AFA Clinical guide lines, pharmacy direct, page: 53
Mims 2003, diseases review, section 4, page 338.
AIDSinfo, clinical guidelines portal, guide lines for the use for
antiretroviral agents in HIV1 infected adults and adolescents,
drugs interactions.

[xv] Science daily, Science news, The many causes of immune
deficiency found on: www.sciencedaily.com/releases/2009/...
Dr Leon Regensberg and Memela M Makiwane(Ed), 2009,
AFA Clinical guide lines, pharmacy direct, page:
[xvi] Foundation for professional development, the integrated of
TB, HIV and STD in the primary health care seting for
doctors, section 1, page 9, Eskom.

[xvii] MedlinePlus, Tuberculosis found at
www.nlm.gov/../tuberculosis.html
Foundation for professional development, the integrated of
TB, HIV and STD in the primary health care seting for
doctors, section 1, page 12 Eskom

[xviii] Patient.co.uk/Tuberculosis found at
www.patient.co.uk>home>professional reference
[xix] Foundation for professional development, the integrated of
TB, HIV and STD in the primary health care seting for
doctors, section 1, page 21, Eskom
Kids health, Tuberculosis found at
www.kidshealth.org>kidshealth>parents>infection

CDC Center for diseases control and prevention, Tuberculosis found at www.cdc.gov/../Itbiandactivetb.htm
[xx] Foundation for professional development, the integrated of TB, HIV and STD in the primary health care seting for doctors, section 1, page 15-24, Eskom

[xxi] Foundation for professional development, the integrated of TB, HIV and STD in the primary health care seting for doctors, section 1, page 73-74, Eskom
www.patient.co.uk/Tuberculosis/investigations

[xxii] Foundation for professional development, the integrated of TB, HIV and STD in the primary health care seting for doctors, section 1, page 73-74, Eskom

[xxiii] Foundation for professional development, the integrated of TB, HIV and STD in the primary health care seting for doctors, section 1, page 75-78, Eskom

[xxiv] Foundation for professional development, the integrated of TB, HIV and STD in the primary health care seting for doctors, section 1, page 83-84, Eskom

[xxv] MedlinePlus, Tuberculosis found at www.nlm.gov/../tuberculosis.html
Foundation for professional development, the integrated of TB, HIV and STD in the primary health care seting for doctors, section 1, page 44-46, Eskom
NHS choices, tuberculosis found at www.nhs.uk/../tuberculosis.html
[xxvi] Dr Leon Regensberg and Memela M Makiwane(Ed), 2009, AFA Clinical guide lines, pharmacy direct, page:14
Foundation for professional development, the integrated of TB, HIV and STD in the primary health care seting for doctors, section 1, page 44, Eskom

[xxvii] University of Maryland, Medical center, pneumonia introduction found at: www.umm.edu>Home>Medical reference>patient education
The New York times, Seach health, Pneumonia adults found at: www.health.nytimes.com>Health> Times Health Guide>p> Pneumonia
[xxviii] Webmd,Lung disease and respiratory health center, pneumonia prevention found at www.webmd.com/../pneumonia/ prevention
Mayo clinic, pneumonia prevention found at www.mayoclinic.com>home>diseases and conditions>pneumonia/Basics
[xxix] MichaelAugenbraum, drugs disease and procedures, pneumonia in immunecompromised patients found at www.emedicine.medscape.com/article18078
[xxx] RHRU, Identification and treatment of minor HIV related infections identified during the course of staging HIV infection, USAID Southern Africa
www.wikipedia.org/wiki/angular chelitis
Chelitis Secrets, The root causes of Angular chelitis and what you can do to stop it found ae www.angularchelitissecrets.com/causes
[xxxi] University of Maryland, Medical center,Candidiasiswww.umm.edu>Home>Medical reference>Complementary medicine
RHRU, Identification and treatment of minor HIV related infections identified during the course of staging HIV infection, USAID Southern Africa
Candidiasis, oral and esophageal, found at www.hab.hrsa.gov>clinical guide>Comorbidities and complications
The Body, Candidiasis Prevention Tips found at www.thebody.com/content/art5867.html
[xxxii] www.wikipedia.org/wiki/herpes zoster

CDC, Prevention of Herpes Zoster found at: www.cdc.
Gov/../rr57e0515a1.htm
MedlinePlus,Shingels found at
www.nlm.nih.gov/../000858.htm
[xxxiii] Webmd, Genital herpes Health Center, Genital Herpes
and HIV found at www.webmd.com../risk-HIV
CDC, Center for disease control and prevention, Sexually
transmited diseases (STD), Genital Herpes-CDC found at
www.cdc.gov/../stdfact-herpes.htm
[xxxiv] Seborrheic dermatitis found at
www.wikipedia.org/wiki/seborrheic dermatitis
MedilinePlus, seborrheic dermatitis found at
www.nlm.nih.gov/../000963.htm

[xxxvi] DermNet NZ, Eosinophilic folliculitis found at
wwwdermnetnz.org?acne/eosinophilic folliculitis
Rosenthal D at al, 1991, found at
www.ncbi.nlm.nih.gov/pubmed.1671328, Department of
dermatology, University of California, School of medicine,San
Fracisco 94143.0506,
Mayo clinic, Folliculitis found at
www.mayoclinic,com>Home>Diseases and
conditions>Folliculitis>Basics.
[xxxvii] MedlinePlus, Fungal nail infection, found at
www.nlm.nih.gov/../001330htm
RHRU, Identification and treatment of minor HIV related
NHS Choices, Fungal nails infection found at
www.nhs.uk/../introduction.aspx